Remembering Alzheimer's

A Husband Bears Witness to His Wife's Caregiving

by

Kevin Lewis

www.VisionSpotsPublishing.com

Copyright Notice

Dedication

To my lovely wife Rebecca of 38 years whom I watched as she cared for me, our family, and her precious mom without missing a beat. She did so without hesitation and with a full measure of devotion. She set an example that I know will serve as a legacy example for our family for years to come.

Contents

Preface

I am humbled that you are reading this work. It has been in my mind for some time now. I felt a nudge from God to pull it out and get it into writing. I slowly began to realize that possibly someone might benefit from what I witnessed and experienced as my wife and I were drawn into a decade long caregiving journey for her precious mom who suffered from Alzheimer's. You don't realize what you have learned from an experience until it is somewhat behind you. It is usually then that you gain perspective and appreciation for what God has taught you through it.

I was originally going to approach this by conducting a great amount of research into the disease, presenting numbers and statistics on how it is impacting families. However, I decided to go a different route and just tell a simple, personal story that is comprised of my observations of my wife in her caregiving role and our experiences through the journey. I realize that it is just one story of thousands.

But my hope is that, through a simple presentation of candid observations and lessons learned, you will hopefully read something that will help you if you are on such a journey.

And, if such IS the case for you, may you experience Our Lord's grace and providence as you navigate the forks, cul-de-sacs, and winding roads that await you. It is a journey that will change you forever, if you remember this:

> *Do not be anxious about anything, but in everything by prayer and supplication with thanksgiving let your requests be made known to God. And the peace of God, which surpasses all understanding, will guard your hearts and your minds in Christ Jesus.*
>
> *Philippians 4:6-7*

Introduction

On the evening of February 6, 2014, I sat at home waiting for a phone call. Earlier that day, I had been sitting with my wife in the nursing home where my mother-in-law, Momma Minnie, resided. We had been notified that she had taken a deep turn for the worse. My wife who had been caring for her for over 10 years went to be with her. I met her there. When I walked in, my dear wife was stroking her mom's arms and hands. After my being with her for a while, she tearfully told me to go ahead home. We knew in our hearts that Momma Minnie was probably not going to make it through the night. So it would be better if one of us would get some rest.

Once I got home, I couldn't settle down. I just sat in front of the TV trying to watch something with my head back, waiting for the call. When it finally came, I heard my wife through her tears say to me "Momma is gone honey. She is gone." We knew this day would one day come. Yet I was still struggling greatly to find words to reassure my wife. I had watched her for over 10 years care for her mom, dutifully…without complaining. The best I could say was "Honey, I'll start calling the family. I'll be right here. Let me know what else you need."

If you've ever gone through the loss of a close family member, you probably know what it means when you hear people say "time just seemed to stop". Everything else takes a backseat while you walk through the process of family notifications, funeral preparation, and the actual service itself.

Being that my wife was the primary caregiver, I had an up-close and personal look at what caregiving for a family member suffering with Alzheimer's looks like. As a Christian, I learned what grace, patience, longsuffering, and other fruits of the Spirit truly look like.

Now that it has been more than two years since her passing, I felt led to take time to capture and share via this book what I learned as a husband and father while bearing witness to my wife's quiet and firm commitment to care for her mom. Care that she gave without seeking attention or notoriety. It is a simple narrative offering personal reflections of our experiences and, more specifically, what I witnessed and learned from this journey.

My hope is that you will glean some helpful insights from our experience.

1: Before It Starts

In the mid-90's, I clearly remember a conversation my wife and I had regarding our parents. We had just buried my dad in November of 1993. It was this event that nudged us to start talking about our parents and the fact that they were aging. It slowly became necessary for us, through the prompting of the Holy Spirt combined with my dad's burial, to discuss what we would do if our remaining parents needed any type of long-term care.

At that time, my mom, stepdad, and mother-in-law were still alive and in good health. But we had seen each of them go through some health battles. Looking back, they were not severe…but I can see now how God used these events along with my dad's death to get our attention about their future…and what our commitments and responsibilities should and needed to be.

We committed to each other that if any of our parents needed care in some form, we would step in and provide it. At the time, we didn't have a clear idea of what that would mean. But knowing that we had made this commitment to each other settled this for us.

Now, let me be clear. I was (and still am, to some degree) the typical driven person who can get somewhat myopic in my desire to achieve things. This

---

Having had this conversation with my wife lifted me out of my career-driven myopia and put me in an accountable position both to her and to God.

---

can be a two-edged sword depending on the situation that one faces.

Being myopic is good when you are focusing on a critical task that needs your undivided attention. It can also be bad when your myopia causes you to be blind to what else is happening around you as you pursue that task.

Having had this conversation with my wife lifted me out of my career-driven myopia and put me in an accountable position both to her and to God. This was vital to our being prepared for what, at that time, we did not know would be awaiting us. I strongly recommend to you now, if you have not had such a conversation, to have it. I cannot imagine what it would have been like if the need to care for my mother-in-law emerged (as quickly as it did, may I say), and we had not even spoken about what to do.

Something that we did not do....which I do regret, is to plan financially. What do I mean by that? First, we should have obtained a healthy insurance plan for her. We were aware of a term-plan that she had. But it was of very low value. As Chris Gardner said in the movie, "The Pursuit of Happyness", this is the part of my life that I called being STUPID. I am using that word intentionally so it will stick. So…don't be stupid. If you are in a situation now, or do anticipate being in the role, of caregiving, begin now to look at the financial picture, particularly life and long-term care insurance.

Naturally, through all of this, it is really important that you and your spouse be on the same page. If the caregiving responsibility does fall onto your exclusive laps, it will shake up your world. Let's be honest. It will change the direction and speed of what is going on in your life. It will have a very significant impact, to say the least.

Prepare for this by growing spiritually in your walk with Our Lord. I have taught Sunday school class for almost 20 years. One point I drive home from time to time is that when some significant emotional event or crisis shows up, you can't go back and fill yourself up with the necessary grace and wisdom that you would have gotten had you been faithful in your spiritual and mental growth. Cultivate your growth now before you have to reach deeper into your spiritual and emotional reservoir.

2: The Phone Call

For us, it was a phone call. It came from my wife's sister. She was frantic and did not know what to do. She had visited Momma Minnie and found her disheveled and speaking incoherently. So my wife took our kids (she was homeschooling at the time) and went down there for a week to see exactly what was happening. To say it was difficult for her was an understatement. To sit in the home she grew up in and see the early effects of Alzheimer's on her own mother was devastating. It became clear to her that we needed to move her in with us.

She returned home and we both came up with the plan to make the move. Up until that time, my precious mother-in-law had not travelled very far from her home. We knew this would be difficult on her, to say the very least. Looking back on this, the actual move and her transition into our home all happened quite fast. At least it seemed that way to me. One confession I do have is that I was oblivious to the emotional toll that this was taking on my wife. One of the wonderful traits I love about her is her strength. She is not a pushover and has tremendous intestinal fortitude. But those traits can also enable one to hide the pain that one is feeling. And that she did. Just because you don't or can't see the pain doesn't mean it is not there. I should have tuned in a lot closer to how this was affecting her.

This pain was coming from several directions. One obvious direction was that of seeing her mom in this condition. It was in sharp contrast to the woman that we remember being outdoors, taking care of her plants and vegetables, serving at her church, and always being ready to receive a visit from a family member or friend. She was no longer in a condition to do so. The great difficulty about this is that Momma Minnie was not aware of this. She could not see any problem. But we could...and we knew there was no turning back.

Another source of pain was conflict with relatives who lived locally to her Momma Minnie but who were not stepping up to help. We never questioned them about this. We just simply felt that it was God calling us to take care of her...even if that meant taking her six hours away back to Virginia. For whatever reason, some of the family accused us of wanting to take control of mom's life. Yet it was they who called us and asked us to step in to help.

Whatever way the word comes to you that your help is needed to be a caregiver, I encourage you as a couple to be prepared to go it alone.

Be prepared for this, should you find yourself in a similar position. You cannot change anyone's mind about what they believe your motives are. Some will deliberately attempt to impugn them. Just be sure that you are following God's leading. This will ensure pure motives on your part.

Whatever way the word comes to you that your help is needed to be a caregiver, I encourage you as a couple to be prepared to go it alone. I am not saying that you should not ask for help. By all means, do so. You want to give family every opportunity to step up. You don't want to look back and have it said that you denied them a chance to help. BUT...don't be disappointed if they don't. And...when they don't, being prepared to go it alone as a couple will only serve you better.

3: The Move

It is all a blur now. We drove down to my mother-in-law's house and started the process of getting her packed up. We did it over a weekend. The physical act of moving was not that significant. What was difficult was staying emotionally stable through everything so as not to cause my precious mother-in-law to become unnerved. She had never lived anywhere else as an adult. Now we were taking her away from everything she knew to someplace that was totally strange and unknown.

Whichever one is serving as the caregiver, the other needs to be tuned in to what is happening to that spouse

I am not sure what we would have done differently. There is one thing that I realize now, looking back, that eluded me at the time. And that is how hard this was on my wife and how marvelous she was in keeping it together while we were in the process of making the move. I know it was all God's grace that made this so. Yet and still, I wish I had had the presence of mind to forthrightly acknowledge this to her at the time. My overriding concerns were the overall logistics of the move and caring for my mother-in-law's house.

My wife's strength is partially rooted in her childhood experiences. She grew up in the segregated south and lost her dad at the age of twelve. She was one of five Black students that integrated the all-white high school in her county in 1965. She developed a needed strength to overcome the obstacles that she faced. Being married to such a woman, it is easy to take her strength for granted. I believe I did that. I was focused on the process, the logic, and accuracy of the decisions we were making. I was not attentive to her emotional well-being.

If I could change anything, I would go back and take time to stop, pray with her, and tell her that I realized how hard this was for her. So, let me say this to you: whichever one is serving as the caregiver, the other needs to be tuned in to what is happening to that spouse. Encourage her, take loads off of her, and think ahead. This will serve you both well.

4: Role Reversal

My wife totally embraced her role in caregiving for her mom. The first few weeks were a bit nerve-racking and, I would say, adventurous. This was the first time in our 25+ years of marriage that Momma Minnie would be staying in our house for a significant period of time. She had her own bedroom and was enjoying being with her daughter and family.

She was still having extended periods of clear-thinking and lucidity, being able to talk about life and family somewhat. But you could certainly see how the dementia was slowly creeping in. What I began to notice was how my wife had slowly, over time, developed habits with Mom that I recall her having with our kids. She helped her bathe, get dressed, helped her into bed at night, read to her. She took time each night to read God's Word to her. One night I peeped in through the door way to see them. I saw this very calm and full smile on my mother-in-law's face. It was the most peaceful I had seen her in many years.

Nonetheless, over the next few weeks and months, the fatigue and stress began to build up in my wife. She never complained. She was totally committed. But it began show. We had two teenage girls going through all of the normal and crazy things that go along with being teenagers. And, we had life itself happening which was pushing all of us into new and unknown territory. What I am not proud of was the myopia I had in not seeing this as clearly as I should have. By that, I mean that I just assumed that my strong wife could absorb and adjust to this. We prided ourselves on being survivors.

We had both been in the Army (that's where we met) and started our lives with great and grandiose dreams. Along the way, we met our Creator personally through His Son Jesus Christ. This new and most vital relationship, looking back now, is what and continues to sustain us.

But your shortcomings don't disappear. They simply show themselves in a different way. For me, my particular shortcoming, in retrospect during these initial weeks and months, was my not being more emotionally in tune with what my wife was experiencing. (I have said this a few times in different ways. I hope it is coming through.)

Looking back, I would have made adjustments to my calendar, commitments, and my pursuits in order to ensure that she and I were staying mentally and emotionally connected. But…that is what God's

16

grace does for you. It fills in the gaps that you don't even know exist.

5: Stress Build-up

Over time, the stress of my wife being at home with her mom each day began to build. My wife now had this day-to-day responsibility to be the physical and emotional caregiver to her mom. It was all new to each of us. New routines had to be developed. New expectations had to be set. New lessons had to be learned at many levels. It is easy in retrospect to look back and see what had to be done and why it was important. But, when you are in the midst of plowing such new ground, you are not able to see everything clearly.

One thing was becoming clear: my dear wife's demeanor began to shift. She was slowly becoming more irritable and impatient. And very understandably so, given that I was causing her to feel isolated by not making efforts to better understand what she was experiencing. This combined with the increasing set of demands on her fed into this. Looking back, I now realize that I was not very tuned in to the additional weight that she was carrying.

It is a blessing from on high to be married to an emotionally and mentally strong woman who complains about nothing. But, that can cause a husband, as it did me, to not appreciate just how

---

This is one of those moments when you want God to speak audibly into your ear and tell you what to do.

---

significant this additional responsibility had become.

Nonetheless, something did happen that got my attention in a huge way. One evening I came home from work and found my wife in the laundry room. As I reached to kiss her, I could see that she had been crying. She does not cry easily. Naturally I asked her if anything was wrong.

STOP! Let's pause right here for a moment. Here I am, coming back into my own house where my mother-in-law has been under the care of my wife for over 1 year at this point. A totally new living situation creating a whole new set of challenges and difficulties – and I am asking her this question. Duh?! I realized very quickly that whatever the issue was, it was 98.2% likely related to concerns over her mom.

I dashed up the stairs to Momma Minnie's bedroom. As I opened the door. She was sitting on the chair with her coat on. She appeared very agitated. She looked up and asked, "Are you ready to carry me back home now? I need to go home". I looked at her bed and it was covered with all of her clothes that she had taken out of the closet and her dresser. This is one of those moments when you want God to speak audibly into your ear and tell you what to do and say. I sat down on the bed next to her and spent the next few minutes trying to convince her that we needed her in our house. That she was vital to being in our home with our family. It was all of God's grace that we were able to calm her down. Slowly I was able to convince her that we needed to put all of her clothing away.

Late that evening, I found out from my wife that this was the most recent in a string of similar occurrences where Momma Minnie had insisted that someone take her back to North Carolina. My wife never told me about those occurrences. But this last one took enough of a toll on her that she just couldn't keep it from me anymore. This was a turning point for me. God had revealed a major blind spot, one wherein I did not or refused to see just how stressful the home situation for my wife in her care-giving role had become. I knew that a change was needed. But what? We were brand new at this and did not have a clue on what other options we might have. Enter God's grace and providence.

6: The Transition to Day Care

One Saturday, we were all outside working on various things around the house. I was in the back cleaning out the shed and my wife was in and out of the house working on our flowers and plants. I came in to get some water and heard the front doorbell ring. My wife, who had just stepped inside to get something came to the door and saw our neighbor from across the street at our front door. She told my wife that her mom was over in her yard. Momma Minnie had walked over there, came into her yard and tried to start a conversation with her. Her husband kept her over there while she came over to let us know. Needless to say my wife dashed over to bring her back.

Have you ever had the shock of a situation hit you slowly? Well, that is precisely what happened here. After we got Momma Minnie back in the house, it slowly hit us just how bad this situation could have turned out. Momma Minnie could have walked off or been hit by a vehicle. However, God saw fit (this is what we choose to believe) to direct her into our neighbor's yard. Certainly we are so thankful that she was safe. But...something else came of this. During the course of the conversation between my wife and our neighbor, we found out that our neighbor's father was suffering from dementia and was participating in a day time care program that got him out of the house during the day. It is known as Adult Day Care. It is a program that provides a location where qualified personnel will provide daytime care to dementia patients.

THIS is God's providence in action. We had no idea this even existed. Had Momma Minnie not wandered over into our neighbor's yard, I'm not sure we ever would have discovered it. We made contact with the local county office and set up a meeting. You've heard the phrase, "this is a God-send". Well, so this was indeed. This program provided a place for Momma Minnie to go each day from 8 to 4:30. She would be a part of a group of people who had various special needs but who were ambulatory and could communicate. They would receive special attention

---

Looking back, I see how God's hand of providence moved in such a protective way to bring us to this phase of needed relief and encouragement for my wife.

---

from a group of professionals trained to care for them. This would also enable Momma Minnie to get out of the house. This last part, I quickly realized, was more important for my wonderful wife who had been taking care of her mom every day for about a year...a very long and trying year.

For the next two years, Mom went to work. That's how she referred to it. In the morning she would tell us she had to get ready for work. In the evening she told us how hard they worked her. One day she complained about the fact that they were not paying her. Not wanting to see her get irritated, we told her that we would make sure she got paid and would pick it up for her. Each Friday evening, we gave Mom some cash. Then she would give it back to us because she wanted to help out with the house expenses. That is how she always was. Wanting to give to us in some way. When she was living in North Carolina, it was vegetables from the garden. Now, it was love from the heart in the only way she knew how.

Looking back, I see how God's hand of providence moved in such a protective way to bring us to this phase of needed relief and encouragement for my wife. Had she had to care for her mom everyday all through her waking hours, I am certain that the effects on her would have been harsh...to say the least.

This is a good place to say something about adult daycare centers. This is a service that is growing in the public and private sectors for those who are suffering from some form of dementia. As a public program, it is not yet available in all states. To find out more about centers where you live, I suggest that you contact your local aging information and assistance provider or Area Agency on Aging (AAA). For help connecting to these agencies, contact the Eldercare Locator at 1-800-677-1116 FREE or www.eldercare.gov. The National Adult Day Services Association is also a good source for general information about adult day care centers, programs, and associations. Call 1-877-745-1440 FREE or visit www.nadsa.org.

7: The Transition to Long Term Care

Recently, I used the term "nursing home" in conversation with a work colleague. She quickly reminded me that the term is now "long term care". It was a reminder that the former term carries a lot of baggage. In looking back, I can certainly recall why that was the case when my wife and I were faced with the reality that it was time to move mom into a facility where she could obtain around-the-clock care.

Mom's heath was deteriorating on several levels. Diabetes became an issue along with other health factors. It was becoming clear that my wife, as much as she wanted to, could no longer give her the care that she really needed at home. But the thought of moving mom into a "nursing home" just tore at my wife. All the questions that you might imagine surfaced. Will she be properly cared for? Will she be neglected? Will the staff be kind to her? Will she suffer abuse?

Naturally you hope that any reputable location providing such services will ensure that the residents are properly cared for. But there is always that nagging thought: "This is my mom. No one will care for her the

---

Your life will shift. You will need to reset your thinking on things, such as your family schedule, obligations, and commitments. This is what service to others entails.

---

way that I will." Nonetheless, we knew that moving her to full-time resident care needed to happen. So we took on the task of finding a place.

We visited multiple locations. Naturally we wanted to find a place that was well maintained, a warm environment, and not too far away. God led us to one that met these conditions. But let me interject one very important point here. My wife was not about to turn her mom over to any place without the staff knowing that she was going to be an <u>engaged</u> caregiver. Intuitively (and, yes...this is a woman-thing), she knew that she needed to stay "in their face" in a friendly, affirming way. This would work to ensure that the staff would give the proper attention to her mom. God help the staff member on duty should my wife ever come in to visit her mom and find out that such was not the case.

A very critical lesson here: your life is going to enter a new and critical season when the long-term care phase begins. Ask God NOW for the grace that you will need should you ever need to travel down this road. Your life will shift. You will need to reset your thinking on things, such as your family schedule, obligations, and commitments. This is what service to others entails. Our home, during this time, went from two to four teenage girls living with us. This came with the arrival of our two nieces whose mom (my sister-in-law) had died of cancer. To say that life was now busier and more chaotic would be a gross understatement.

My wife, God bless her, was a wife, mom, caregiver, custodial parent, and household manager, just to name the obvious roles. If there is something that I would have changed, if I could turn back the clock, it would be that I would have worked harder at trying to anticipate her needs. I would have worked harder at seeing things through her eyes.

Another turning point in my mindset came when I went with my wife on a visit to see her mom. I usually did not go with her on her visits as she would be engrossed in addressing some personal hygiene items, which were time consuming. And given everything else that was happening in our home, having one of us stay back was usually the better choice. I remember walking through the lobby and going into the special wing where dementia patients resided.

On this particular visit, I had been there before…but it had been awhile. As we walked through the lobby, we stopped as my wife spoke with a staff member. While she was doing so, I looked around and

---

As Paul Newman said in the movie "Cool Hand Luke", I got my mind right.

---

saw some of the residents sitting in wheelchairs. One was on the younger side. She caught my eyes and said, "Are you here to see me?" I smiled and nervously looked away.

Later, as I was sitting in the room watching my wife care for her mom, it dawned on me just what a saint I was married to. As Paul Newman said in the movie "Cool Hand Luke", I got my mind right. Many residents in these facilities are essentially abandoned by their families. My lovely wife visited her mom once or twice a week. She felt it to be her God-given duty to be by her mom's side until one of them was called home by God. The selfish part of me naturally wanted that to be her mom. And eventually it was. Her mom finished her earthly race to join her Savior with my wife sitting by her side.

8: Finances

No matter how prepared you may think you are when it comes to money, this will always be a very difficult area for most families. In looking back at this, particularly in the days and weeks after my mother-in-law's passing, I realized that there were some basic things that we should have done at the onset when my wife's caregiving responsibilities were starting to take shape years before.

First, be sure to review your family member's finances. Get a good handle on their assets. This is important as these assets will come into play should

---

Be sure to review your family member's finances. Get a good handle on their assets.

---

you ever have to move your family member into a long-term care facility.

Second, ensure that a will and advanced medical directive are in place. This is where it can get quite difficult. And…this is a place that I hurt the most for my wife when we took the necessary actions to get this done. Some of my wife's siblings were not totally on board with what we were doing for her mom. In fact, it got quite ugly with some of them. We discovered that some thought we had some hidden agenda when it came to getting these legal documents in place. I believe their reactions were rooted in guilt on their part. Nonetheless, be sure to get this done.

My wife kept her cool throughout this time. She did shed tears a time or two (that is an understatement). But she remained committed to what she felt God called her to do for her mom. I could use some scriptures here to describe her. Suffice to say that she simply stayed faithful to the commitment that we had made many years back to care for our parents should any of them needed us. And that is what she did. It was a demonstration of commitment quietly in action.

Third, be sure to review what life insurance is in place. That is not a comfortable topic to address, but it is indeed important. Get professional help when doing this. There are many factors involved here which will impact the type and amount of insurance you will need.

Suffice to say, much information is available today that addresses sources of financial assistance for Alzheimer patients and their caregivers. The link below from the National Institute on Aging will serve as a good starting point for finding out what these sources are and how they can be pursued.

https://www.nia.nih.gov/alzheimers/faq/are-there-any-sources-financial-help-people-alzheimers-or-their-caregivers

9: Kids

At the time that we moved my mother-in-law into our home, we had our two teenage daughters with us. A year later, after my sister-in-law's death, we took custody of her two daughters so they could live with family instead of becoming wards of the foster care system. So I was

---

It's easy to let kids get somewhat self-absorbed. And, we can even make excuses for them by trying to "protect" them and to keep their lives "normal".

---

living with six females, a great adventure...to say the least. When people would ask me what life was like living with all of "those women", I was quick to say, "Well, I can always easily find my underwear when looking in the dryer."

It was a memorable time...and a very difficult time. I watched my wife be a caregiver and a new custodial parent while also continuing to be a wife and mother. Let me be very honest here: it was nothing but God's grace that we did not lose our two daughters during this time. I was immersed in running a multi-national non-profit, traveling internationally as well as domestically. When I was not traveling, I was chasing other business opportunities which took my mind away from what was going on at home.

I can write a whole other book on just this one part of our time with mom living with us. Let me just offer a few reflections, should you have minor children in your home while serving as a caregiver.

First, don't forget about them. Make sure you set aside time with them that takes them away from the caregiving environment that they have found themselves in. Looking back, I realized that our daughters and nieces did not have the time to get mentally and emotionally ready for this strange environment that they would find themselves in. As far as they were concerned, it just happened.

Second, make sure you give them the opportunity to vent. The normal stresses of school and relationships don't go away. They will need somewhere to open up. When they do, do NOT minimize or blow off how they feel. Yes…inside you will be thinking "Come on…is this really that important?" Well…YES…to them it is. Their frame of reference is much smaller and governed by an obviously immature mindset. That is not their fault. It is simply reflective of their own reality. If I could have changed something during this time, it would have been to be more patient with them.

Third, get them to take whatever weight you can off of the caregiver. I recall how may wife worked so hard to juggle our household. I remember a conversation we had one evening where all she could think about was getting the "next item" on her list checked off. What might be a series of mundane, simple tasks can turn into a cumulative set of tedious burdens. I learned what a relief it was for my wife if someone would simply vacuum, clear out the sink, or fold the clothes in the dryer. The list goes on. This may seem so obvious, but let me say that spreading out the household tasks among the kids will pay dividends in many ways, not the least of which is that the burden becomes lighter and the tedium starts to dissipate.

It's easy to let kids get self-absorbed. And, we can even make excuses for them by trying to "protect" them and to keep their lives "normal". But…if you are caregiving, this is the <u>new normal</u> for your home. If the kids help to pick up some of the slack, downstream in their own lives they will become more appreciative for what you taught them and for the ethic that you passed on.

10: My Spouse and Her Family

As I have said several times, looking back at the years that my wife was taking care of her mom, I simply took for granted the commitment she was living up to. I reflect on that time now and see a wife who loved her mom and was going to do what needed to be done. It was indeed a lesson in witnessing someone doing tedious tasks with a loving, uncomplaining spirit. It was also evidence of how she had grown in her faith and how she desired to make her faith real.

One particular emotional component that we endured during these years was the anger and ridicule that she bore from one of her sisters. I saw it as guilt. Seeing my wife care for her mom as she did served to make this particular sister angry and accentuated the guilt that her sister felt. She had lived much closer to my mother-in-law but, when it became obvious that she would need more care, my sister-in-law did not step up to the task. I believe that she was in denial of what was happening to Momma Minnie. I can understand that. Nonetheless, she could have chosen

---

No…it was better to simply ignore and absorb.

---

to be supportive, but chose not do so. In fact, she made it her mission to malign my wife to other family members.

There were several times that I wanted to pick the phone and put my sister-in-law in her place. Yes…I thought about it…a lot. But I am thankful that I did not do that. It was all of God's grace and the Holy Spirit that intervened. What would I have accomplished if I had done so? What would the environment be now amongst family members if I had sunk unto that type of behavior?

No…it was better to simply ignore and absorb. And, it has paid off….with unexpected blessings. Other family members have since told us in recent months just how much they admired and appreciated what we (really what my wife) did for Momma Minnie. They have apologized for not being more encouraging. This goes to a lesson that my wife and I learned long ago: we must be prepared to do what God has called us to do without expecting to receive any acknowledgement or recognition on this side of heaven. That is how you maintain a peaceful mindset as you journey through where God is taking you. And that is how you build a legacy of humble service that your children and grandchildren will not forget.

11: Lessons to Take Away

This decade of my seeing my wife serve as her mother's caregiver taught us both some lessons. Most, if not all, are sprinkled throughout this story. Nonetheless, I thought it would be helpful if I put them all in one place for your reference:

- Have the conversation NOW about what you will be prepared and committed to do should a caregiving need in your family arise
- Cultivate your spiritual and emotional growth now before you have to reach deeper into your spiritual and emotional reservoir
  - As a Christian, that means prayer, deep conversation with your spouse about the mutual challenges you have faced thus far, your victories, and what you learned from them
  - Pray together at least once a week

- ○ Read God's Word and other books that address practical Christian living
- Plan financially, medically
  - ○ At minimum, make sure that the person for whom you are caring or might care for is properly insured
  - ○ Ensure that a will and advanced medical directive are in place
- Once one of you enters the day-to-day caregiving role, be prepared to be Gumby (remember him?)
  - ○ Being flexible and agile are the minimum requirements for the caregiving journey
  - ○ Remember: it will be a new season and a new normal for your family
- Be prepared to go it alone
  - ○ You will likely have family members make verbal commitments to help only to later find out that they are absent when needed
  - ○ This will likely be the case for you
  - ○ Accept it
  - ○ Yes...ask for help but don't be surprised if the help does not come
- Encourage your spouse DAILY
  - ○ Don't take it for granted that he/she knows that you appreciate him/her
- Develop an anticipatory mindset
  - ○ Be proactive in getting ahead of the need curve in your household by staying on top of basic chores
  - ○ DON'T PROCRASTINATE

One last point: NEVER forget that your family, friends, and others whom you don't even know are watching. How you handle the stresses, tensions, problems, sweet moments, all of that, will bear witness to your faith...how deep and how meaningful it is to you.

When your family is standing over your grave, what will they remember about how you handled this family member who slowly deteriorated before everyone's eyes?

I can say with great peace that my lovely wife met the call and was a blessed daughter to her mom up until Momma Minnie passed into the Lord's hands. Was she without fault or error? Of course not. We are flawed human beings with shortcomings as well as gifts. What I want to leave you with is that I witnessed a wife, mother, and daughter do what was called upon her to do without reservation. As she cared for her mom and her family, she endeavored to live the fruit of the spirit. I wish I had realized it as much then as I do now.

Let me encourage you to pursue such a course, whatever your role may be in the caregiving journey. It will indeed be worth it.

About the Author

Kevin Lewis is an author, publisher, and life coach. As of this writing, he is serving as the principal for a Christian school in Alexandria, Virginia.

He has served as a military officer, defense contractor executive, and consultant. He also has served as a Sunday school teacher, trustee, and deacon board chairman for his church where he became a Christian.

He has been married to his wife Rebecca for 38 years. They have five children and six grandchildren. Without the Good Lord and his wife he would be a mess living in darkness.